Road Accidents to Children

The Role of the NHS

Heather Ward

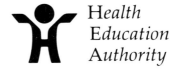

Health
Education
Authority

© Health Education Authority, 1991

ISBN 1 85448 224 6

Printed by the KPC Group London & Ashford, Kent

Acknowledgements

Preventing Road Accidents to Children – the Role of the NHS was a project commissioned by the Health Education Authority from the Child Accident Prevention Trust (CAPT).

The project was supervised by a joint team. Karen Ford and Christine McGuire, from the HEA; Barbara Sabey, the chairman of CAPT's Professional Committee, and Michael Hayes, CAPT's Technical Officer. The project was carried out and the report written by Heather Ward, whilst she was at the Transport Studies Group, University College London. The help and enthusiasm of all those on the project team, who provided input and suggestions at all stages, and all those consulted, is gratefully acknowledged. We are also grateful to Jerry Read of the Department of Health and Gavin Lord of the Department of Transport who commented on the final draft, and Jenny Fieldgrass who edited the manuscript. The final document was prepared for publication by the HEA.

The Health Education Authority is grateful to the Institution of Highways and Transportation for permission to reproduce the diagram on page 32 from *Guidelines for Urban Safety Management* (IHT, 1990).

Contents

Foreword		vii
Summary		ix
The Role of the HEA		xi

1. Introduction — 1

2. Background to the Road Accident Problem — 4

3. Review of Research, Practice and Materials — 8
1. Review of road safety research undertaken by the Department of Transport — 8
2. Accident studies — 10
3. The need for, and use of, good data — 12
4. Engineering — 13
5. Education, training and publicity — 14
6. Enforcement and encouragement — 20
7. Requirements for further research — 21

4. Review of Current Links and Activities — 23

5. The Role of the Health Service in Reducing Road Accidents Involving Children — 28
1. The NHS as a provider of information — 28
2. The NHS as a provider of personnel and expertise — 30
3. The NHS as an educator — 37
4. The role of the Director of Public Health — 38

6. Pointers for Action — 41
1. The Department of Health — 41
2. Regional Health Authorities — 41
3. District Health Authorities, directly-managed units and NHS Trusts — 42
4. Family Health Service Authorities and general practitioners — 43
5. The Health Education Authority — 44
6. Conclusions — 45

References — 46

Appendices
1 People consulted by the project — 50
2 Groups who attended one-day seminar at CAPT — 53
3 Useful addresses and resources — 54

Foreword

The consultative document *The Health of the Nation* published in June 1991 suggested that the span of healthy life of the people of England could best be improved if attention were concentrated on a few key areas. Quite rightly, one of the areas proposed was the prevention of accidents. These are a major cause of death and serious ill-health. In 1990 more than 5000 people died on the roads in England. Far too high a proportion were children. About a quarter of all deaths among schoolchildren are caused by road accidents and this figure represents about two-thirds of all accidental deaths among children of school age.

These tragic facts led the Department of Health in 1990 to invite the Health Education Authority to examine the role the National Health Service could play in the prevention of road accidents to children. We joined with the Child Accident Prevention Trust in setting up a special project team to carry out this task. This report is the result of over a year's hard work.

I urge all those in the NHS who have a role to play in tackling this problem to study with care Chapter 6 'Pointers for Action'. This sets out clearly and succinctly the contribution each authority can make. For our part, we in the HEA will be paying close attention to the questions addressed to ourselves. It will be our aim to give effective support to the actions of our colleagues in the NHS.

In this field, as in every other, in the words of *The Health of the Nation*, achievement of improvements requires a shared commitment from all those with responsibilities for health. I am confident that this report will inspire the commitment needed.

Sir Donald Maitland
October 1991

Summary

Road accidents are a major cause of death and injury to children. In 1990, over 48 000 children were reported to the police as injured in road traffic accidents in Great Britain. In addition there are known to be large numbers of accidents, particularly involving pedestrians and pedal cyclists, that go unreported to police despite involving injury.

The pattern of accidents varies between different parts of the country and between towns as a result of use of different means of transport. Boys tend to be injured more often than girls and the 11–15 age group is involved in more accidents per 100 000 children of this age than are younger children. The older children tend to have most of their accidents on busy residential and main roads and are more at risk on the way home from school than on the way there in the morning. The very young children tend to be injured within two hundred metres of home on minor residential roads.

One important characteristic of children's road accidents is that they do not cluster at locations on the road network and, as they are diffusely scattered, they are difficult to treat using traditional traffic engineering measures. The report outlines recent important advances in the field of road safety engineering, including the introduction of 20 miles/h zones.

The importance is highlighted of well-researched and properly targeted education, training and publicity programmes as a way of changing behaviour. Three areas where significant changes have taken place are in the introduction of Children's Traffic Clubs in the eastern region of England, the development of new material for inclusion in the National Curriculum, and the integration into it of existing material.

The European office of the World Health Organisation, within the context of Health for All 2000, and the Secretary of State for Transport have both set casualty reduction targets to be met by the year 2000, and it is within the context of these targets that much of the current work is being undertaken.

Four influential reports have led the way in recognising the need for the National Health Service to work together with local authorities and other agencies to set and achieve common objectives for reducing road accidents involving children. The initiatives aimed at reducing children's road accidents are many and varied, some are systematic and well recorded, others are local projects with little institutional support. The cost of road accidents to the country and to individuals is high. There is no easy and inexpensive solution and many programmes will not yield quantifiable results for some time to come. The report recognises that whilst there are many competing health demands at all levels, it is the Department of Health that sets priorities and allocates resources. *The Health of the Nation* (1991) has shown that the Department of Health *can* take the lead in recognising that road accidents *are* a health issue. What is needed now is the development of a policy framework for road accident prevention that will allow those in the health authorities to explore ways, through their contract and service agreements, to reduce injuries to the children for whose health they have responsibility. The Health Service has itself much to gain from fewer casualties resulting from road accidents.

This report identifies the specific roles of the Department of Health, Regional and District Health Authorities, the Health Education Authority and other agencies within the health structure. In particular it highlights the need for the Health Service at various levels to provide information, personnel and expertise, to act as an educator and through the central function of the Directors of Public Health to act as advocate to identify needs and co-ordinate action.

The Role of the HEA

The HEA is a special health authority within the National Health Service, whose mission is to 'ensure that by the year 2000 the people of England are more knowledgeable, better motivated and more able to acquire and maintain good health'. While the HEA plays a strategic role in advising the Secretary of State for Health, it also provides information and advice about health to the public. It works to support other organisations, health professionals, and indeed anyone who provides health education directly to members of the public.

The HEA is committed to joining with others to prevent road accidents to children, and has fostered links with the two key voluntary agencies in the field: the Child Accident Prevention Trust (CAPT) and the Royal Society for the Prevention of Accidents (RoSPA). The HEA is keen to see concerted efforts made to prevent child accidents, covering material and environmental hazards as well as health education, and involving a whole range of statutory and voluntary organisations, together with central and local government.

In its Operational Plan for 1991–93, the HEA undertakes to develop and publicise local approaches to child accident prevention. In 1991 two new resources were produced in collaboration with the key government departments and voluntary agencies involved in child accident prevention: the Approaches to Local Child Accident Prevention Project, and *Preventing Accidents to Children: a Training Resource for Health Visitors* (details of both are given in Chapter 4). In addition, the theme of accident prevention continues to be covered in other appropriate resources the HEA produces such as the *Pregnancy Book* and *Birth to Five*, both of which are given free of charge to all first-time parents in England.

In 1992, the HEA will also be supporting the 'Play it Safe! – Action for Child Safety' campaign. 'Play it Safe!' aims to promote the prevention of accidents to children within the UK through a series of national and local activities, and to lead to permanent improvements in children's safety. A major part of the campaign is an 8-week BBC TV series to be shown from

January 1992, and repeated throughout the year. To support 'Play it Safe!', the HEA is producing a 12-page leaflet on all aspects of child safety, including road safety. As with all HEA materials, this leaflet is being pre-tested prior to publication.

The 'Play it Safe!' campaign will maximise the opportunity offered by the TV series, provide national promotion and support for practitioners, promote multi-disciplinary, cross-agency activity; provide national publicity, materials and other support as a framework for local activities; and encourage evaluation at national and local levels. It is being co-ordinated by the Child Accident Prevention Trust in conjunction with the BBC, RoSPA, BSI, the Home Office, the fire services, and the four national health education bodies. Campaign staff will provide resource materials, arrange meetings and facilitate contact between people planning child safety measures.

1 Introduction

The government department that has the principal
responsibility for leading the way in road accident prevention
and casualty reduction is, and has always been, the
Department of Transport (DTp). Its document, *Children and
Roads: a Safer Way* (Department of Transport, 1990*a*) sets out the
government's strategy for reducing the number of child
casualties on our roads. That document outlines the problem,
reviews what steps are currently being taken to reduce the
number of casualties and provides a 'framework and focus for
action by the many agencies, organisations and individuals'
who can contribute to this reduction. It recognises that the
Department of Health and the Department of Education and
Science each have a key role to play in the prevention of
children's road accidents.

Following publication of *Children and Roads: a Safer Way* in
1990, the Health Education Authority (HEA) was invited by the
Department of Health (DH) to carry out a special project to
consider just what the NHS's role should be in terms of
preventing road accidents to children. The HEA set up a
project team, and commissioned the Child Accident Prevention
Trust (CAPT) to undertake a thorough review, consult with
specialists inside and outside the NHS, and to come up with
recommendations on new ways of working within the
reorganised NHS.

The structure of this project

The assessment of the role of the NHS began with a review of
current research, publications and materials at a national level
and, where possible, a local level. Interviews were conducted
with Health Service personnel to try to determine the level and
effectiveness of present initiatives being undertaken within the
NHS. Current links were examined between road safety officers
and Health Service personnel in the context of prevention of
children's road accidents. Discussions were also held with
specialists from the Department of Transport, Department of

Trade and Industry (DTI), DH, local highway and health authorities, academic research groups, individual researchers and various national bodies with an interest in child safety. Those consulted are listed in Appendix 1.

Following these discussions the project team and a small group of specialists met with the aim of identifying areas in which the Health Service could make a contribution, both in the short term and longer term, to the reduction in the number of road accidents involving children. Those who took part in this one-day seminar in January 1991 are listed in Appendix 2.

Aside from the work described above, three other important and influential documents form the basis for this study. The first is *Action on Accidents: the Unique Role of the Health Service* (National Association of Health Authorities, and Royal Society for the Prevention of Accidents 1990).* In this report a joint NAHA/RoSPA strategy group set out four general objectives:

- to outline the scale and nature of the accident problem and its consequences for the Health Service
- to identify the agencies responsible for accident prevention and specify the nature of their responsibilities
- to review current knowledge, attitudes and activities related to accident prevention in the Health Service
- to develop an outline strategy for the health service, at the same time identifying possibilities for collaboration with other agencies.

This present study takes account of the objectives and recommendations of the NAHA/RoSPA report in relation to action on road accidents involving children.

Secondly, *Basic Principles of Child Accident Prevention: a Guide to Action* (Child Accident Prevention Trust, 1989), which aims to raise awareness of the child accident problem in general and to present first steps in starting a prevention programme.

Thirdly, *The Local Authority Associations Road Safety Code of Good Practice* (Association of County Councils *et al.*, 1989), which underlines the importance which local authorities attach to the reduction of road casualties. It aims to channel the enthusiasm of local authorities in a more effective way and

* Now known as NAHAT, National Association of Health Authorities and Trusts.

recognises that local and other authorities without highway powers have a role to play in support of road safety both directly through their various services and indirectly through influencing public opinion.

The authors of these four documents urge co-operation in setting up multi-disciplinary groups to pool knowledge, expertise, data and resources with a clear remit for action by each agency represented.

The first part of this report contains a review of current research, practice and materials together with a brief overview of links that already exist between local and health authorities. The second part of the report draws upon the discussions with specialists and explores ways in which the Health Service can contribute to the reduction in road accidents involving children both through its own efforts and through co-operation with other agencies.

The Health of the Nation

This report appears shortly after the publication of the Department of Health's consultative document, *The Health of the Nation* (1991), which raises the issue of health promotion at a national level, confirms that road accidents to children are a health issue, and agrees that preventing them is an important part of health promotion.

The HEA hopes that apart from opening up the debate, stimulating new initiatives and new ways of working, this report on the contribution the NHS can make will provide key personnel within the Health Service – particularly those involved at district level, and those involved within public health – with real ideas on how further to develop and expand their work on preventing road accidents to children. The HEA will be pleased to receive feedback on this report.

2 Background to the Road Accident Problem

In every class of 30 schoolchildren, two of these can expect to be injured in a road accident before their sixteenth birthday. Road accidents are a major cause of death and injury to children and the 417 fatalities recorded in 1990 represent more than 60 per cent of fatalities resulting from accidents of all types involving children aged 15 years and younger (Department of Transport, 1991).

In 1990 over 48 000 children were reported to the police as injured in road traffic accidents in Great Britain, of whom nearly 23 000 were pedestrian casualties, a further 9000 were pedal cyclists and over 14 000 more were car occupants. In addition there are known to be large numbers of accidents particularly involving pedestrians and pedal cyclists that go unreported to the police despite involving injury (see Chapter 3, section 3 'The need for, and use of, good data').

About 1 casualty in 5 is killed or seriously injured when all modes of travel are taken together, but when pedestrians are

Percentage of child casualties in 1989 by mode of travel – all severities

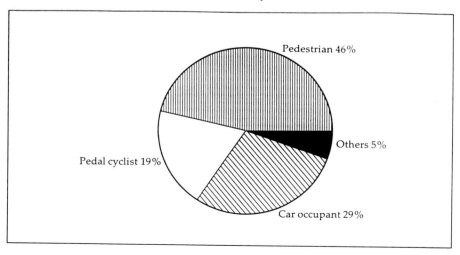

considered by themselves, one-quarter are killed or seriously injured compared with about 1 casualty in 6 for pedal cycling and 1 casualty in 9 for car occupants. Not only are children more likely to be injured as pedestrians, they tend to be injured more seriously than cyclists or car occupants.

Numbers of child pedestrian casualties per 100 000 children are about 2.5 times the number of adult pedestrian casualties per 100 000 adults. Within this composite rate are marked differences between age groups and modes of transport, as illustrated below.

As children become older, their mobility increases and the amount of adult supervision decreases. They travel further to school and venture further afield to play and to take part in leisure activities. As they grow older they tend to cycle more. These casualty rates tend to vary between different parts of the country and between towns as a result of the use of different means of transport. Climate and topography contribute to a tendency for cycling accidents to be more prevalent in the south of the country whilst those involving pedestrians occur more often in the north. These differences mean that authorities in each part of the country need to be aware of local and regional factors that may influence accident occurrence.

Child casualties in 1989 by age and mode of travel – all severities

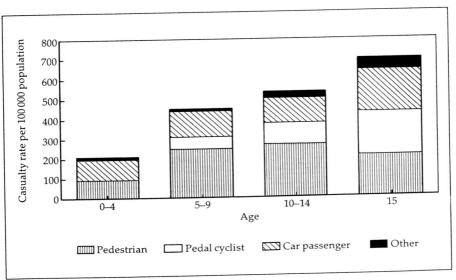

Besides differing from region to region, and from free-standing towns to metropolitan districts, the numbers and proportion of accidents involving children differ from one part of an urban area to another. In town centres there are large concentrations of traffic and pedestrians and it is here where clusters of pedestrian accidents occur but these rarely involve children. Once away from town centres, on the main routes and in the residential areas, accidents of all types tend to be more scattered and it is in these more suburban areas where children are over-represented in pedestrian and cycling accidents relative to their numbers in the population. Very young children tend to be injured on local roads near to where they live, whilst older children have an accident pattern more like that of adults, occurring more often on main roads. Recent studies in Birmingham (Lawson, 1990) have highlighted a particular problem of a different injury pattern in inner city areas.

Children are vulnerable on their way to and from school. Tight (1987) found that in the five towns he studied, the percentage of child pedestrian accidents occurring on such journeys ranged from 19 to 33, the risk being about twice as high within $\frac{1}{2}$ km of the school as further away, and higher on the way home than on the way to school.

In general, nearly 60 per cent of fatal and serious child injuries occur between 3.00 pm and 7.00 pm, covering the times during which school journeys are made as well as other play and leisure activities. Children are also more likely to be injured during good weather and in the summer months, most likely reflecting their greater exposure as they tend to stay outside longer. Boys are injured more often than girls and in the 11–15 age group they are involved in twice as many accidents as girls as pedestrians, and in nearly three times as many accidents on pedal cycles as girls of the same age (Mills, 1989). As car passengers, however, the rates are about the same.

The picture that is emerging of child pedestrian and cycle accidents is that the 11- to 15-year-olds is the group most often injured, especially boys. These children tend to have most of their accidents on local distributors and main roads and they are more at risk on the way home from school than on the way there in the morning.

The very young children, those under 5 years of age, tend

to be injured on residential streets within a few hundred metres of home and nearly always as pedestrians rather than cyclists.

Perhaps most importantly, children's accidents do not cluster at locations on the road network and as they are diffusely scattered they are difficult to treat using traditional traffic engineering measures.

Local highway authorities have recognised that the child accident problem in particular, and the pedestrian and cycling problem in general, cannot be tackled piecemeal and new important initiatives are being taken which recognise the need for inter-agency co-operation both within local authorities and between local health authorities.

Casualty reduction targets

At a national level the Secretary of State for Transport set a target in 1987 of a reduction in casualties by one-third of the mean 1981–85 level by the year 2000. This has been translated into regional and local targets and it is within this context that local highway authorities are working in the 1990s.

The World Health Organisation (WHO) has also set casualty reduction targets of one-quarter of fatalities resulting from accidents by the year 2000 and Regional and District Health Authorities are working towards this through the Healthy Cities Network (now called the UK Health for All Network) and other initiatives. The health authorities also recognise the need to work together with other agencies.

Local highway authorities and the police have clear statutory obligations to improve the safety of the roads in their area. The health authorities have a duty to assess the health needs of the population and the rest of this report will be aimed at exploring ways in which, and to what extent, the NHS has a role to play in the prevention of road accidents and reduction of casualties to children and young people under 16 years of age.

3 Review of Research, Practice and Materials

Recently several researchers and the Department of Transport have published extensive reviews of road safety research and materials. This study highlights some of the more important advances and collates a selection of recommendations for further research and action.

1. Review of road safety research undertaken by the Department of Transport

A major review of pedestrian safety research was undertaken for the Transport and Road Research Laboratory (TRRL) by Heraty (1986) who reported on a wealth of information on pedestrians of all ages over a wide range of topics, under the following headings:

accident statistics and studies
traffic management and environmental design
vehicle design
pedestrian behaviour
exposure and risk
perception and attitude studies
education and publicity
legislation and enforcement.

The rest of this chapter will highlight developments since the publication of this report.

A general observation made by Heraty was that there was a lack of integration between research areas which was hampering progress in understanding the causes of accidents and the nature of the problem. She also highlighted a lack of knowledge about the effectiveness of measures introduced to reduce pedestrian casualties. More specific recommendations included:

• more in-depth and sharply focused on-the-spot studies of

pedestrian accidents to examine specific aspects of the accidents and actions leading to them

- more detailed inter-regional comparisons and analysis of police accident data with their relationship to accident data held by hospitals
- more understanding of the effect on accident occurrence of vehicle speeds, road layout and alignment, parked cars, and other traffic and environmental management issues
- siting and use of crossing facilities together with other factors such as time of day and traffic flow to determine factors affecting pedestrian risk
- conspicuity of both pedestrians to drivers and of vehicles to pedestrians
- risk to children aged 10–14 years with the need to understand their accident pattern together with behavioural and perceptual issues
- studies into whether increased perception of risk leads to safer road-user behaviour
- the need for more education programmes to be developed.

Heraty's report contributed to the government's review of pedestrian safety undertaken during the second part of the 1980s. In 1987 the Department of Transport published *Road Safety: the Next Steps*, which was the result of an inter-departmental review of road safety policy in which the government recognised the need to set targets for casualty reduction. In 1987 the Secretary of State for Transport announced that a national target had been set of reducing the number of casualties by a third of their mean 1981–85 level by the year 2000. At the same time more funding for research into road-user behaviour was announced together with the setting up of a road-user behaviour unit at TRRL. Vulnerable road-users, especially children, were a high priority. The consultation document, *Pedestrian Safety: New Proposals for Making Walking Safer* (Department of Transport, 1989), set out priorities for action in the following areas:

education and training
traffic calming and accident prevention road engineering being seen
pedestrian and driver responsibility
research to identify further ways of reducing pedestrian casualties.

A further consultation document was issued in 1990 which was to become widely circulated and influential in raising people's awareness of the child road casualty problem. This was *Children and Roads: a Safer Way* (Department of Transport) already referred to in Chapter 1. *Children and Roads: a Safer Way* provides an excellent summary of the work being carried out by the Department of Transport and this, together with projects being undertaken by other government departments, local authorities, national and voluntary organisations, the Health Education Authority, academics and consultants, is reviewed briefly in the rest of this chapter.

2. Accident studies

The Scottish Development Department (SDD) commissioned the MVA Consultancy to undertake a study of child pedestrian accidents and road crossing behaviour in Scotland (Scottish Development Department, 1989). Some of the major findings of this report were:

- most children in Scotland do not cross the road in the way they were taught
- the general standard of road sense and behaviour is poor
- running across the road and not looking for traffic are the most common features of child pedestrian accidents.

Specific findings of interest which are in line with earlier work are that boys were injured twice as often as girls, and that children with impaired eyesight or hearing are over-represented in the casualty figures by as much as 30 to 1. Children from homes where the head of the household is in a semi-skilled or unskilled job, or are unemployed (groups D and E), are also over-represented in the casualty figures. The study also found that when children were accompanied they were involved in fewer accidents. On the road environment side, children were injured on roads with parked vehicles, faster traffic and at junctions. The report recommends:

educational measures to
    improve basic kerb drill
      give guidance on crossing among parked cars
      target young boys to reduce running across roads
      develop timing and co-ordination skills

engineering measures to
  reduce speed of traffic
  improve parking provision to aid crossing the road,
    particularly at specially narrowed points
  introduce measures to deter crossing at dangerous sites
promotion of accompaniment to
  encourage adults to accompany children
  encourage children to seek supervision
  make drivers more aware of unsupervised children.

Lawson (1990) provides an up-to-date review of other research and accident studies and makes a major contribution to the subject with his report, *Accidents to Young Pedestrians: Distribution, Circumstances, Consequences and Scope for Countermeasures*. This work was commissioned by the AA Foundation for Road Safety Research and was carried out using data for Birmingham. One of the important features was its use of records of HM Coroner in Birmingham. This allowed a detailed study to be made of fatal accidents to young pedestrians over a five-year period. These records were supplemented by means of postal questionnaires and interviews with seriously injured casualties. The study found a disproportionate number of casualties involving children under 10 years of age from Asian families and children from lower social groups. In findings which correspond to those of the Scottish study and a study of contributory factors in urban road traffic accidents (Carsten *et al.*, 1989), it was found that about 20 per cent of the pedestrians admit to not looking before crossing and half of the pedestrians said they did not see the vehicle before being struck by it. Many drivers did not see the pedestrian until it was too late to take avoiding action.

Among Lawson's recommendations are that

- methods of education, training and publicity should take specific note of the characteristics of those at risk and the fact that they are often the least receptive to, and least able to assimilate, the road safety message
- more research is needed to evaluate road-user behaviour of pedestrians of different ethnic origins
- statements about the effect of traffic and transportation policies on accidents to young pedestrians, casualty reduction targets and options for countermeasures be included in local authority road safety plans

- measures to reduce volume and speed of traffic and to restrict inappropriate parking should be introduced.

3.   The need for, and use of, good data

Lawson's study highlights the need for good data. Recent studies by TRRL have investigated the extent to which accidents involving injury on the highway are under-reported to the police and hence do not appear in the police accident data (STATS19). Tunbridge (1987) used the hospital in-patient data for Scotland (SHIPS) to match the STATS19 data to study the relationship between the nature of injury and accident circumstances. About 70 per cent of the records matched and these data were used to investigate, among other types of injury, patterns of injury to child car occupants where it was found that injuries children sustain when unsecured in cars are predominantly to the head. Further work was carried out in Oxfordshire (Tunbridge *et al.*, 1988) to assess the severity of injuries on a clinical basis and the degree of under-reporting. This study highlighted the low proportion of injury accidents involving pedal cyclists that were reported to the police. Studies of injury patterns such as these by Tunbridge are important as they enable an assessment to be made of need for changes in vehicle design, the extent to which restraint systems reduce injury and the resulting change in severity and location of injury brought about by such restraint systems and changes in vehicle design. These studies also highlighted the need for pedal cyclists to wear helmets if head injuries were to be reduced. Mills (1989) studied pedal cyclist accidents linked with hospital data and found that where no other vehicle was involved, almost none of these accidents was reported to the police. Even when a motor vehicle is involved, under-reporting rates can be as high as 50 per cent for slight injuries. There is a third database which holds information on some pedal cyclist injuries and this is run by the Department of Trade and Industry (DTI), who have responsibility for leisure accidents. The database is Leisure Accidents Surveillance System (LASS) and holds sample hospital data on pedal cycle accidents where no motor vehicle is involved. (See Department of Trade and Industry, published annually.)

The studies reported here highlight the lack of an integrated database in which all casualties are recorded. Such information would allow injury patterns to be researched better, leading to development of more effective vehicle design, restraint and protection systems. The levels of under-reporting that have come to light suggest that total road accident costs are being significantly underestimated.

4. Engineering

In recent years the research emphasis has been to find ways of reducing accidents on urban roads especially where children are involved. These accidents tend to be scattered over the road network and the most promising engineering solutions are based on the designation of a hierarchy of roads within a town in which main roads for through travel are identified. The remaining roads are regarded as residential and appropriate engineering measures may be introduced to reduce the speed and volume of traffic. It is important for drivers to be aware that they are in a residential area, that local roads are seen as places where people may meet and not feel threatened by traffic travelling at inappropriate speeds. To help identify ways in which a safer environment may be achieved, TRRL undertook a major research project where roads in residential areas in five towns were adapted to make them safer. The approach demonstrated that the most scattered accidents can be reduced by as much as 10 per cent by introducing inexpensive engineering measures as part of an area-wide strategy to reduce accidents (Mackie *et al.*, 1990). Early in 1991, the government authorised the use of 20 miles/h speed limit zones in residential areas and these, implemented as part of an urban safety management strategy, are seen as an important step forward in reducing child casualties (Institution of Highways and Transportation, 1990). To help local authorities establish these zones and implement local area safety schemes, a proportion of the Transport Supplementary Grant* has been allocated for this purpose.

One of the findings from the five-town Urban Safety

---

* A grant from central government to the highway authorities formerly for schemes on main roads only but now allocated for local road schemes as well.

Project was that by altering the parking arrangements (whereby isolated parked cars were encouraged to park in bays sheltered by building out the kerb to reduce the road width to be crossed by pedestrians) accidents involving injury to pedestrians were substantially reduced (Mackie *et al.*, 1990).

By the application of traffic management and traffic calming techniques in local areas, both the safety and environment can be enhanced. This is especially important in the parts of towns and cities where there is a higher than average occurrence of child accidents which often corresponds with older, terraced types of housing with little or no off-street parking and few safe places for children to play. Although these schemes are expensive and wide ranging in their effects, they can lead to immediate reductions in accidents, help to make people feel safer and bring about environmental improvements.

5. Education, training and publicity

(a) Education

The Road Traffic Act 1974 gives local authorities responsibility to provide road safety education and training for young people. In 1982, Singh undertook a wide ranging review of pedestrian education and mass media communications programmes. This section lists major developments since then. More recently, studies of road safety education have been undertaken by Singh and his colleagues for TRRL which have identified the lack of a structural foundation upon which traffic education could be based (Singh and Spear, 1989). Few schools had a policy for implementing a traffic education programme. In general, no teacher had overall responsibility for traffic education, although such a teacher was recommended, possibly as part of a wider responsibility for personal social health and safety education. With the introduction of the National Curriculum this situation is starting to change.

Teacher training programmes were also reviewed (Spear and Singh, 1989) with the conclusion that few institutions included road safety education but most did include health education courses. Spear and Singh recommend that teacher training courses could include road safety education as part of health education. Another deficiency that was identified was a general lack of awareness among teachers of the resources available for road safety education.

These findings have encouraged TRRL to lead the development of a Code of Good Practice in Road Safety Education Within Schools (Harland *et al.*, 1991) in parallel with the Local Authority Associations Road Safety Code of Good Practice, which urges local authorities to relate educational programmes to local circumstances and the development of a co-ordinated programme of education. The TRRL guidelines suggest 'ways in which authorities and schools can organise themselves to deliver a coherent and effective course of road safety education to their young people and monitor its progress.' These guidelines have been developed by a working group comprising representatives from teachers, education and health advisers, and road safety officers.

A pilot study to test the code of good practice has been set up by the Department of Transport in conjunction with the Department of Education and Science. The authorities taking part are Sheffield and Hertfordshire (Harland *et al.*, 1991). Singh and his colleagues are assessing the effectiveness of the project for TRRL.

The introduction of the National Curriculum provides opportunities for road safety education to be integrated into the school curriculum. The National Curriculum Council (NCC) has produced and issued to all schools Curriculum Guidance 5: *Health Education*, which places safety as one of the nine components in a framework for a health education curriculum for children between the ages of 5 and 16. The safety component is stated thus:

> 'The acquisition of knowledge and understanding of safety in different environments, together with the development of associated skills and strategies, helps pupils to maintain their personal safety and that of others.' (National Curriculum Council, 1990)

The NCC also stress that the relationship between a school and the local community is important, as well as developing programmes in conjunction with parents, governors and families. The HEA is currently consulting the Department of Transport with regard to undertaking joint work with school governors.

Aspects of safety education can be incorporated into

foundation subjects of the National Curriculum even where no specific reference is made. An example would be the use of road accident statistics and surveys in mathematics or their analysis and presentation using computer techniques in technology. Issues in road safety could form the basis for exercises in English and environmental aspects could, for example, be covered in geography. Examples of this cross-curricular approach are given in Curriculum Guidance 5.

An example of the material the HEA produces is *Health for Life* (Williams *et al.*, 1990), which is a two-volume health education programme planning and classroom activity guide for primary-school teachers. There is a large section on 'Keeping Myself Safe' which includes using the roads with special reference to school journeys. Other material produced for schools by the HEA is listed at the end of this report.

Many of the techniques and materials recently developed have been for use with the National Curriculum. TRRL and the British Institute for Traffic Education and Research (BITER) have developed, with sponsorship from Texaco, *Secondary Steps*, a resource in road safety activities for use in personal and social education (BITER, 1990). RoSPA has produced, with the help of SPAR, *Streets Ahead*, for 7- to 11-year-olds. This is a four-module pack providing ideas and resources for an integrated safety education programme with National Curriculum attainment targets for the core subjects (Royal Society for the Prevention of Accidents, 1989). Nottinghamshire County Council have developed AT/TERMS (Attainment Target – Traffic Education Resource Matching System), which is a computerised catalogue of existing road safety materials that are each matched to attainment targets and levels of the core subjects of English, mathematics and science (see Singleton and Woodcock, 1990). The system is most appropriate for use in junior and primary schools.

Extensive resource lists have been provided by the National Centre for Road Safety Education at the University of Reading for use with children aged 3–7 years, 7–11 years and for lecturers and teenagers in further education colleges. These resource lists are referred to in Appendix 3.

The importance of integrating local examples into the taught road safety material is stressed by all authors. An important part of this exercise is the co-operative development of safer routes to school. Several research projects have been undertaken which collect information by questionnaire from children at schools to ascertain their daily route to school (Tight, 1987; Road Safety and Design Partnership, 1988; Towner *et al.*, 1990) in order to assess risk and exposure and to develop routes using less busy roads or easier places to cross. Autoglass have sponsored a Safe Journey to School award which encourages schools to set up projects to find ways in which the journey to and from school can be made safer.

Pre-school children are vulnerable both as pedestrians and as car occupants. At this young age the material and initiatives are aimed at raising the awareness of parents to their responsibility in setting a good example to young children, in choosing somewhere safe for them to play and in teaching them about traffic.

One major initiative which was launched in 1990 is the Children's Traffic Club, sponsored by General Accident Insurance Company, in the eastern region of England. The club provides parents with materials and teaching aids to help them to develop road safety skills in their young children. The Children's Traffic Club is based on a Scandinavian model which has been very successful with claims being made of up to a 40 per cent reduction in casualties in Norway. Each child, from their third birthday, receives an initial pack of materials. The parent or guardian registers the child who then receives material at six-monthly intervals until their fifth birthday. Family Health Service Authorities (then Family Practitioner Committees) mailed out the first packs to the children in their records aged 3 years. The materials were developed by TRRL, who are monitoring and evaluating the project, which includes an assessment of where the children live (by postcode) obtained when a parent responds to the initial pack (see General Accident, 1990). General Accident are committing £1 million over a five-year period.

Street-wise Kids is an older club that operates in London but on a smaller scale than the Traffic Club. There is interest in other parts of the country but the initiative is beyond the means of a local authority.

The Tufty Club is older and different in nature with a squirrel providing the role for good road behaviour. These materials were developed by RoSPA and evaluated by Firth (1973). A more recent evaluation (Antaki *et al.*, 1986) found that children who had been exposed to the Tufty Club material did not show higher levels of knowledge than their peers and like Firth found that this knowledge did not generalise to the road situation. Ampofo-Boateng and Thomson (1989) cite research findings which indicate that printed material may increase knowledge but not affect behaviour on the road.

(b) *Training*

Children and Roads: a Safer Way (Department of Transport, 1990*a*) presents an up-to-date review of training programmes for children of all ages as pedestrians and cyclists. Work in the universities of Strathclyde and Edinburgh (Ampofo-Boateng, *et al.*), has indicated that conventional road safety training such as the Green Cross Code may not be the most appropriate method and has demonstrated that young children can be trained to find safer places to cross and to acquire appropriate visual information to help them cross busy streets. More work needs to be done in this area but the results from the early work look promising. Its major drawback is that it needs a package of practical training to be developed for adults to use with small groups of children. However, table top models are currently being developed which should reduce the resources required. Again there is the ever present problem of how to reach the more vulnerable children.

Children with special needs require more specialised training procedures and materials. The MVA consultancy study of Scottish pedestrians highlighted the accident involvement of hearing-impaired children. Some existing materials for use with children with special learning needs are to be found listed in Appendix 3 but a greater understanding of their needs is required in order to produce even more appropriate materials.

Cycling is very popular among children. Younger children tend to be involved in accidents whilst playing, travelling too fast or just falling off (Mills, 1989). Older children use their bicycles for travelling further, for paper rounds and for journeys to school. This age group is more likely to be struck by another vehicle. Breeze and Southall (1990) undertook a survey of the behaviour of teenage cyclists at T-junctions from video films of riders. The study concluded that whilst nearly all those observed rode their bicycles with confidence, less than half appeared to be paying attention to riding safely but more did so with increasing density of traffic and with age of cyclist. Breeze and Southall suggest that the high level of confidence observed might be the result of education and training strategies but these same strategies may not contribute effectively to imparting roadcraft skills. The study recommends that a defensive riding scheme should be considered and that as much emphasis should be placed on roadcraft as on learning prescriptive rules.

General experience indicates that cycle training undertaken in school playgrounds or parks does not transfer well to the road situation. Training should be well supervised on roads where possible, even though it requires greater manpower resources.

Seeing and being seen are important elements of keeping safe. The relationship between conspicuity and speed is complex but any way in which a driver's attention can be drawn earlier to a young pedestrian or cyclist might give sufficient time to slow down, take avoiding action or even stop. Texaco have recognised the importance of the use of reflective and fluorescent materials on children's clothing, bags and bicycles, and have launched a campaign called Children Should be Seen and Not Hurt. Stickers to aid conspicuity have been issued through their filling stations. The problem with wearing reflective material, similar to that found by proponents of cycle helmets, is that children do not want to look stupid in front of their friends. A task facing educationists and trainers is to change attitudes, especially children's, to make conspicuity and safety aids more acceptable.

(c) *Publicity*

Research in this area indicates that whilst visual methods of instruction including videos, films and slides can hold the interest of a child, the evidence for their effectiveness is far from clear. Children tend to remember important parts of a road safety message when a media personality is featured (McGarvie *et al.*, 1980), but Singh (1982) concludes that there is no convincing evidence for changes in everyday behaviour. One of the more successful series was Willy Whistle, where crossing between parked cars was one of the behaviours targeted. Accident reductions and behavioural changes were noted.

Ampofo-Boateng and Thomson (1989) cite examples of the use of videos and suggest promising avenues to explore. One might be the production of videos highlighting dangers in children's own localities and their use as feedback for children's road crossing behaviour.

Publicity campaigns often rely on posters and leaflets. There is little evidence to suggest these have more lasting effect and promote a change in behaviour. However, multi-media campaigns properly targeted can be effective. The Department of Transport is to set up campaign planning teams together with road safety officers and others involved (Department of Transport, 1990*a*). The HEA provides posters, leaflets and books as part of its health promotion activities. The HEA distributes the material of other groups, such as the Child Accident Prevention Trust, as well as its own. Two major publications aimed at parents are the HEA's *Pregnancy Book*, which mentions the need for an in-car infant carrier, and *Birth to Five*, which contains a section on safety including child restraints in cars and referring to the Green Cross Code. (Both books are given free to all first-time parents.) However, more information about what children are capable of, in developmental terms, when crossing the road is needed. The HEA's leaflet for the forthcoming 'Play it Safe!' campaign contains this type of information.

6.   Enforcement and encouragement

Enforcement of road traffic law by the police is an important element in maintaining and improving the safety of roads. Perhaps the laws most relevant to the safety of children are those covering:

observance of speed limits and traffic signs, and the wearing of seat belts and child restraints.

Whilst it is difficult for the police to prosecute all offenders in residential areas because of the practicalities of manpower resources and judgement about policing policy, it is important that an enforcement policy is part of a wider strategy for casualty reduction. Many police are community based and can help encourage drivers, riders, pedestrians and parents to take action to work together towards greater safety for an area.

Encouragement by people other than the police is important especially in the use of a car seat appropriate to the size and weight of the child, that is properly secured and properly used.

Encouragement is important for children to wear cycle helmets, undertake cycle training and wear reflective clothing.

The Local Authority Associations Road Safety Code of Good Practice recognises the importance of encouragement of safe driving practices amongst all employees, of maintaining public and school transport to the highest standards of safety, of improving targets for road accidents involving their own vehicles, discouraging drinking and driving at all functions and of making maximum use of their influence in support of road safety promotion.

7. Requirements for further research

Many of Heraty's 1986 recommendations have been translated into research projects and when all the research initiatives are taken together, there is a substantial body of work in progress. Whilst not all of it is directed specifically at children much of the research into accident reduction for the vulnerable road-user groups is applicable to children as well as adults.

Heraty's observation that there is a lack of integration between research areas still holds in 1991 although at a practical level integration is urged by the Local Authority Associations in the *Road Safety Code of Good Practice* (Association of County Councils *et al.*, 1989) and by the Institution of Highways and Transportation (1990) in its *Guidelines for Urban Safety Management*. The Child Accident Prevention Trust (1990) also give practical ways of working together. However, although NAHA/RoSPA (1990) provide a framework there is no research to provide guidance on how these partnerships could proceed in the prevention of road accidents.

The 1990s will see the introduction of local area safety schemes incorporating 20 miles/h zones and traffic calming techniques but there will be failures, not because the engineering techniques are unsound but because there is little knowledge of how to consult communities on road safety matters that directly affect them and require them to balance safety with ease of accessibility.

Lawson (1990) and the MVA Consultancy (Scottish Development Department, 1989) both point to the need for more studies in road-user behaviour of young pedestrians. Much work in road-user behaviour is being undertaken, especially in Europe. Rothengatter and De Bruin (1988) review much of the work in this area but the behaviour of different ethnic and social groups is not covered. Much of the work in the road-user behaviour area is directed more at education, training and publicity (ETP) than at the development of engineering solutions to reduce children's accidents.

Many authors highlight the lack of proper evaluation of ETP programmes but gradually more information on effectiveness has become available. The three areas in which significant change has taken place are in the introduction of the Traffic Club in the eastern region of England, the development of new material for inclusion into the National Curriculum and the integration into it of existing material.

Ampofo-Boateng and Thomson (1989) identified two areas needing further research. One is how to make the best use of popular road safety films for children by proper targeting. The second is to explore the use of video films at a local level to feed back to children their own behaviour. This is a common training method with adults especially in the area of sales and public speaking. It is also used extensively in sports coaching.

The work being carried out at Strathclyde and Edinburgh universities appears to have potential but more funding and research are needed to produce a training product that can be used by parents or teachers.

At a local level is an area of research that is only just beginning to emerge as important. This is to develop programmes for the community for use through schools and other focal points to ascertain their needs and priorities and where among them safety lies. Roberts (1991) is attempting to address the question of how it is that most parents manage to keep their children safe most of the time, even in difficult circumstances, and what can be learned from them. This research is being conducted in a housing estate in Glasgow's southside working with a parents' action group and is being carried out in association with Smith of Edinburgh University. More research of a sociological nature is required in the field of children's road safety – the problem is too complex for purely engineering or educational solutions.

4   Review of Current Links and Activities

During the course of this study several links at a local level were discovered. These were mainly where a road safety officer had contacted an individual in the Health Service or vice versa. Very little work of a structured nature was discovered except for the TRRL project in Sheffield and Hertfordshire (Harland et al., 1991). Several people had reported that multi-agency groups had been set up but many of them had foundered because of lack of leadership and institutional commitment. This present study was conducted on a short timescale and it has not been possible to undertake a systematic review of links and activities, but the study has drawn upon interviews with personal contacts and the work of Benson in the Approaches to Local Child Accident Prevention Project (ALCAPP) which has been undertaken by the Child Accident Prevention Trust supported by the HEA and DTI (Benson, 1991).

Approaches to Local Child Accident Prevention Project (ALCAPP)

The aims of ALCAPP were to:

offer information on the methods, resources and skills
needed to bring down local accident rates
act as a manual of good practice
act as a contact point and network for local practitioners.

Local and health authorities and voluntary organisations were asked to supply information about child accident prevention work that they carried out, including road accident prevention work. Information from over 200 local areas was assembled and studied.

Besides finding out about current initiatives, Benson reported on the difficulties of inter-agency working such as lack of data, difficulties in assessing the effects of interventions, and lack of sophistication in joint working. Lack of national and local political priority has meant that there is no policy framework in place. This in turn leads to a low level of resources being allocated to accident prevention work in general.

Benson found that in the field of road accident prevention quite a lot of the work at a local level is being carried out in isolation by groups unaware of the existence of current work being carried out by others, even within the same authority. Energy is spent by groups organising 'safety days' where road safety is only one aspect. The input into these days is often unresearched and material is used because it is easy to prepare or is already to hand. Little or no evaluation is undertaken of the impact of these campaigns as no targets have been set nor objectives clearly defined.

ALCAPP produced a number of resources which provide ideas and skills for local practitioners from a range of backgrounds who are involved in accident prevention, including:

- *Planning for Effective Action – Working Papers for Local Group Activity*, which looked at inter-agency working, setting up and running groups, attitudes and approaches to child accident prevention, getting access to relevant information, and undertaking a programme of work and evaluation.
- *A Checklist for Effective Working*, which provides those working on local child accident prevention initiatives with a quick checklist of the important questions that need to be answered, if the work is to move forward smoothly and successfully.
- *Who's Who in Child Accident Prevention*, which provides a cross-referenced alphabetical listing and description of the jobs to be done by those most commonly involved in local child accident prevention (CAP) work, together with a description of the departments and agencies in which they work.
- *A Practical Approach to Evaluation*, which aims to help make sense of a confusing and jargon-filled subject and to provide some pointers for local CAP practitioners wanting to incorporate evaluation into their work without a lot of fuss and mystification.

There is also a *Summary and Discussion of the Project's Work and Findings*, which provides a brief overview of ALCAPP and discusses the picture that emerges of contemporary CAP work going on in local areas. There are other short booklets: *An*

Integrated Approach to Road Safety: Plans and Progress within one Highway Authority – how Oxfordshire County Council has brought all involved much closer together, and *Home Safety Equipment Loan Schemes*, a case study which looks at the experience of Bristol in getting child safety equipment to families on low income.

ALCAPP was not simply a research project. The intention was that the project should also try to create better contact between local child accident prevention practitioners, and much of the information gathered about local work is now stored on the ALCAPP database, housed at the 'Play it Safe!' campaign headquarters. The database allows easy retrieval of information about local contacts and the kind of work they are engaged in. During 1991, CAPT, supported by the HEA, has also run a series of training seminars around the country on both ALCAPP and *Preventing Accidents to Children: a Training Resource for Health Visitors* (see below).

Healthy Cities

Still at a local level, but more cohesive, are the Healthy Cities programmes, set up, or inspired by, the European office of the World Health Organisation (WHO) in 1987. Now known as the Health for All Network, these groups have done much to bring people together but even these have tended not to have given road accident prevention a high priority. Most local authority highway engineers are unaware of the Health for All 2000 targets and projects.

Car seat and cycle helmet schemes

Most successful local initiatives have focused on car seat loan or helmet purchase schemes because these are areas where people can see the product of their efforts, the sale or loan of equipment which can be counted and reported on. But the statistics show that car occupants make up only 16 per cent of the killed and seriously injured child casualties reported. Whilst the car seat loans are important, they will not go far enough towards solving the problem even if all children are properly restrained. A similar point could be made for the wearing of cycle helmets. The real problem is child pedestrian and pedal cyclist casualties, whether or not there is a head injury. But little is being done by multi-agency groups to target and prevent accidents of these types, probably because the problem is much more difficult, needs specialist knowledge, is more expensive to treat and does not give results that can easily be quantified.

Training professionals – *Preventing Accidents to Children: a Training Resource for Health Visitors*

The training needs of professional groups are now being recognised as needing multi-agency input. *Preventing Accidents to Children: a Training Resource for Health Visitors* is a pack that has been developed for both initial and in-service training of health visitors. It can also be used by school nurses, nursery nurses, and parent groups. Published by the HEA in 1991, and funded and developed by a group comprising the HEA, DTI, Child Accident Prevention Trust, Health Education Board for Scotland (HEBS), Community Education Development Centre (CEDC) and the Northern Ireland Department of Health and Social Services (NIDHSS), the pack aims to increase the awareness of health visitors of the concerns of families and children about accidents, and to stimulate a review of current child accident prevention practice in the clinic and in homes. It is also designed to increase knowledge and awareness of accident risk and causation and of appropriate prevention strategies.

The pack comprises a tutor's guide (*Preventing Accidents to Children*), which contains materials for group work based on activities and discussion points, a set of black-and-white photographs and an interactive video. It is available from the HEA.

The research study on which *Preventing Accidents to Children* is based (*You Can't Watch Them Twenty-four Hours a Day*) is published separately, and is available from CAPT (Combes, 1991).

Pointers for further working

The child accident problem is complex and multi-agency working – with links both at local and at national level – is necessary. However, it will only work when there is leadership, a clear remit for action by each group, organisational commitment and continuing support, together with an understanding by group members of the different tiers of the different organisations and roles of the professionals who work within them.

The greatest scope for achieving targets and objectives will be by working together to:

- set up information systems which will allow inter-regional and national comparisons, and systems for local information such as the one being developed by Walsh and Jarvis in Newcastle upon Tyne (see Chapter 5)
- share information between community health services, Family Health Service Authorities (FHSAs), Directors of Public Health (DPH), road safety officers, road safety engineers, planners and police with objectives defined and leadership agreed
- produce educational material for schools. The TRRL project will be a model for this type of work when the results of evaluation are known
- produce input into health promotion materials including the planning and evaluation of effective campaigns with public health, community health, the highways department and health promotion officers being represented
- enable the community to identify its own road safety needs in terms of feelings of safety for its children and in improving the safety of the local roads. Such a group will work to enable the community to participate in the design of schemes which go a long way to meeting their needs.

A code of good practice needs to be developed for working together to set and achieve common objectives within different organisational structures and constraints.

5 The Role of the Health Service in Reducing Road Accidents Involving Children

Earlier chapters have set out the background to the child road accident problem, briefly reviewed some of the recent research, described some of the initiatives, and sketched the types of links and co-operation found during the course of the study. This chapter aims to draw from those preceding it, and from a one-day discussion meeting of specialists, to present a case for a structured and committed role for the NHS in the reduction and prevention of road accidents involving children.

1. The NHS as a provider of information

According to the Department of Transport figures, road accidents to children cost the country nearly £450m in 1989 (Department of Transport, 1990b). This figure includes an allowance for treatment and social costs. Whilst good data are a basic requirement for any accident prevention programme, whether it be education, enforcement or engineering, they are also the basic requirement for resource management.

S. Walsh and S. Jarvis are currently undertaking a study in which information on childhood accidental injury is being registered at the Department of Child Health, University of Newcastle upon Tyne. Data are being collected from coroners' inquest files, hospital in-patient admissions, a 20–25 per cent sample of attendances at accident and emergency departments and police data on road traffic accidents. Besides collecting basic information on age, sex and place of residence, information will also be collected about type, location and severity of injury, socio-economic factors and treatment given with an assessment of outcome. Information such as this should provide the health authority with valuable information about where to deploy resources and should, especially if shared with the local highway and education authorities, target vulnerable groups more effectively.

At a local level, a Resource Management Initiative computer system is gradually being introduced into hospitals. The accident and emergency department element of the system may not be introduced so rapidly. It should enable detailed information to be obtained about how many people of different ages and sex are treated, what resources were needed for their treatment, which areas are most in need of further attention, and assessment of savings in health care from accident prevention programmes. A recent TRRL report provides costs of long-term disability resulting from road traffic accidents (Tunbridge *et al.*, 1990). Accurate data inform decisions at all levels of policy making and strategy development so without data the setting of, and progress towards achieving, national and local targets for accident prevention cannot accurately be assessed. Not only are data used to determine scientific validity of countermeasures, they are essential for developing models of good practice in community development, in changing the perception of safety both of individuals and groups and in bringing informed pressure for change to bear at both local and national levels.

The Health Service 'has a unique role to play because of its ability to generate, interpret and disseminate accident information' (National Association of Health Authorities and Royal Society for Prevention of Accidents, 1990). Health information should be shared with other authorities such as highways, planning, education and police. In this the accident and emergency departments have a role to play in installing databases which provide information useful to these other groups. Databases such as the one being developed by Walsh and Jarvis could aid the co-ordination of data across authorities. Whilst it is recognised that co-ordinated accident databases on regional and national scale are an ideal for longer term implementation, much could be done today without the need for extra resources if accident and emergency departments extended their system of notification of attendance by children under 5 years of age to cover all children who had been involved in a road traffic accident. Not all accident and emergency departments notify liaison health visitors, or others, of children's attendance at hospital, and of those that do, few provide casualty slips for those over 5 years of age.

Within the data gathering exercise the NHS has implemented Hospital Episodes System (HES) which has replaced its hospital in-patient enquiry (HIPE) scheme. HES is a 100 per cent sample of in-patient data across the country and this, together with its relatively recent implementation, will in time offer a database from which information on casualties of road accidents can be extracted. As part of its HASS and LASS initiatives, the DTI is about to pilot a scheme in conjunction with the Department of Transport to collect road accident data. If this proves to be feasible, its implementation could be a way of collecting data of known quality by others than the Department of Health. This type of partnership could be supported by health authorities and Trusts whilst a national scheme to record all attendances is set up in every accident and emergency department. Although there is some overlap in the collection of in-patient data, the two systems fulfil different data requirements.

The Health Service could do more to help Traffic Clubs by either collaborating with respect to providing name and address data according to age to local highway authorities or by committing resources to aid the dissemination of the Traffic Club material.

2. The NHS as a provider of personnel and expertise

(a) Contribution towards and support for local highway safety and environmental schemes

Arising from the targets of the WHO-inspired programme, Health For All 2000, many health authorities are promoting Healthy Cities initiatives of which accident prevention is a part. There is a body of evidence pointing to the greater health needs of the poorer neighbourhoods and some health authorities are beginning to target their resources on such neighbourhoods.

In parallel, and somewhat in isolation, research on the transport side is indicating that it is these same neighbourhoods that are experiencing greater than average occurrence of road accidents, especially those involving children. (See for example, Lawson, 1990.)

The general picture from the highways side is that local highway authorities are beginning to tackle the more difficult to treat accidents by implementing local area safety schemes which often incorporate traffic calming measures such as road humps and narrowed sections of road. Since January 1991, 20 miles/h zones have been approved by the Secretary of State for Transport. Because measures to reduce speed and volume of traffic in residential areas have much further reaching effects than engineering schemes at individual sites, these programmes should be integrated with other initiatives being taken in the area. Local area safety schemes only work effectively if the help and co-operation of local people have been enlisted in setting the agenda for problem specification, design, implementation and use, as some people will inevitably suffer some inconvenience in travelling to and from their homes as they may have to take a slightly longer route or travel more slowly on certain roads. As engineering measures for road safety move into the streets where people live rather than being a feature of main roads more people's daily lives and travel patterns will be affected. As safety becomes a concern of the community all professionals involved must work together, in ways such as those shown in the diagram overleaf, to improve the quality of life for the people who live in these areas. It is here that the community health services, the Family Health Service Authorities, the health education and health promotion units, encouraged and supported by the Regional and District Health Authorities, have an important role to play.

In the first instance the areas with the highest child accident problem are likely to be those with older housing, probably inner city, where the housing stock will be owned by the local authority or by private landlords. There will be a fairly high density of housing with little off-street parking and few safe places to play. The road network is likely to have a high number of junctions, many of which will be crossroads and afford opportunity for drivers not resident in the area to take short cuts through it.

The role of the Health Service here is to provide the other part of the picture, that of the health needs of the people who live in the area described by the highway authority in terms of land use, traffic flow and accident statistics. This will lead to a better understanding of the problems in the area, of which road safety is only one. A safety strategy can only be developed when the problems are understood. A road safety scheme in a local area is unlikely to be accepted by people whose housing conditions are inadequate unless the two are improved as part of an environmental package. It is here that the Director of Public Health and the community health services have an advocacy role to play to bring all sides together to improve the quality of life in which the road environment plays an important part.

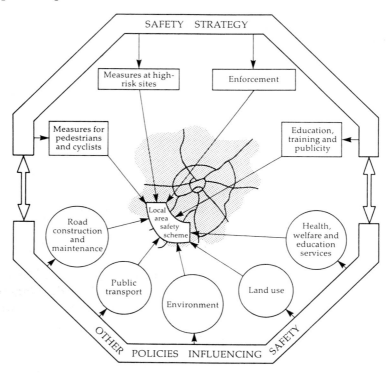

SAFETY   STRATEGY

Measures at high-risk sites

Enforcement

Measures for pedestrians and cyclists

Education, training and publicity

Road construction and maintenance

Local area safety scheme

Health, welfare and education services

Public transport

Environment

Land use

OTHER   POLICIES   INFLUENCING   SAFETY

SOURCE: IHT (1990)

Once a scheme is designed, preferably with input from all relevant professionals and representatives of the local people, the role of education, training and publicity at a local level becomes important. Here health visitors and those from Family Health Service Authorities have a role to play in disseminating information to help people understand the changes and teaching them how to use the local roads more safely. If safe routes to school have been introduced, knowledge about their need and use are vital if safety benefits are to follow.

For safety schemes to work, the local community needs to feel it has been involved in the design and that the people have some control over their environment. It is here that the Health

Service has the skills to communicate with the local people and with other groups in local authorities such as the police, road safety officers and engineers, housing and environmental health officers, planners and architects, and the education authority.

(b) *Contributions of specific groups within the NHS*

(i) *Community paediatricians.* The accident statistics reveal a peak in road accident occurrence between 3.00 pm and 7.00 pm during weekdays. This is made up of children being injured on their way home from school together with accidents occurring once the child has reached home or wherever they will spend the time until a parent or older brother or sister returns. The consultant community paediatrician is in a good position to identify areas where there is a high level of latch-key children. From accident and emergency department casualty slips, where schemes to collect them exist, they are also in a position to monitor the occurrence of injury arising from road accidents both in high risk areas and in the health district as a whole. The consultant community paediatrician can fulfil a monitoring role and be proactive in identifying, for example, the need for safe areas to play and increased provision for after-school care, especially for younger children. There is a need for dialogue and action with social services, housing, planning and highway safety departments of the local authority.

(ii) *Midwives* are in an influential position to encourage good practice from birth onwards in safe carriage of children in cars and to explain the importance of close supervision of toddlers near roads, both busy and quiet. The midwife should be a good source of advice on car seat loan schemes, purchasing, installing and correct use.

(iii) *Health visitors* are in a good position, like consultant community paediatricians, to identify problems within a community both in accident occurrence and in feelings of safety as expressed by members of the community. With changes in the Health Service, there is a shift away from home visiting as routine so the potential for opportunistic one-to-one counselling has diminished, but advice on road safety matters, both to individuals and small groups, could be dealt with at the health centre or clinic.

Within the community the health visitor has a signposting role and it is important that they be well informed as to who can help the community with problems and concerns relating to road safety. Often the health visitor does not know who is responsible for road safety matters nor what their remit is. As part of a multi-disciplinary group it could be the health visitor's remit to work with individuals or groups from the community to explore their concerns and to help them identify their needs. They then have a role in acting as a focus for stimulating action whether it be to press the local highway authority to act or to press for joint action to design acceptable safety schemes once the highway authority has initiated the process based on an analysis of accident and other information.

Some health visitors also receive casualty slips from accident and emergency departments but often feel there is insufficient information on which to base an analysis to lead to coherent action. Better links with road safety officers and sources of health education information would enable health visitors to play a wider role in improving the safety of children.

Health visitors see children at about their third birthday so could at that time enquire whether the child had received a pack from a Traffic Club, if one were operating in that area. They could also enquire about use of car seats and provide additional information to that already provided by midwives about loan schemes, purchasing and installing. As the child gets older and starts to cycle, training and the wearing of a cycle helmet could be advocated.

(iv) *School nurses and doctors.*   Once the child goes to school, responsibility passes from the health visitor to the school nurse who monitors the health of children through school. Again, they are in a good position to identify changing trends in type, severity or location of accidents, some of which may be unreported to both police and hospitals. The training and publicity function of school nurses and doctors in relation to road accident prevention is potentially more than at present, and their roles could be developed by dedicated training and the provision of good, relevant written material such as posters and leaflets prepared jointly with input from the local health education/health promotion unit and road safety officer.

(v) Family Health Service Authorities and general practitioners. The new GP contract recognises the role the GP has in health promotion and accident prevention. *Action on Accidents* (National Association of Health Authorities and Royal Society for Prevention of Accidents, 1990) recommends that FHSAs incorporate accident issues into their practice annual reports and that they identify community needs. The report also recommends that the accident prevention content of child surveillance programmes be developed in conjunction with the community health services.

The general practitioner has the opportunity to take a much more active role in the community by working more closely with the District Health Authority or Trusts in identifying specific road accident problems, jointly establishing targets and strategies, collecting and disseminating material and advice, and being supportive of action taken by the local authority. Some examples of action that could be taken are as follows.

- Under the new GP contract arrangements there is provision for payment for holding health promotion clinics. At present this only covers specified subjects. Advantage could be taken to promote road safety including giving information on local initiatives and loan schemes and giving advice on feeling safe and keeping safe on the roads. But the FHSAs, through their contracts with GPs, would need to recognise these types of clinic.
- Waiting rooms provide an opportunity to display health promotion material. This should include road accident prevention materials which can be informative posters and leaflets together with innovative material such as toys, games and videos. Research has shown that these could provide promising results especially if relevant to the local situation. For GPs, however, they would need commitment to accident reduction to encourage them to purchase the necessary equipment and materials when the gain is longer term.
- The FHSAs in the eastern region of England have already co-operated with the local authorities in disseminating Traffic Club materials. More FHSAs could co-operate and even commit resources to enable this scheme to be introduced in other parts of the country.
- Road accident prevention material could be incorporated into

patient held records with advice given according to the age and development of the child.

All five groups together with others involved in primary health care can help to improve the safety of children with special needs. This group includes children with behavioural difficulties as well as those with mental and physical impairments. Specialist teaching in road safety is needed for these groups which requires the development of materials tailored to their needs. Children with hearing difficulties are particularly vulnerable and need to be identified. Understanding the particular difficulties faced by these children is an area in which the community health services and the general practitioners have a role to play in feeding in information to those who will develop the programmes and materials.

The primary health care services have a role to play in helping to get the road safety message to those most at risk. They also can have an important input into identifying those most at risk. Health Service professionals are in a unique position in having a range of face-to-face contacts with those in higher risk groups. They already tend to be working in areas of our towns and cities which have poorer health and safety records than other parts. Although more research is needed in this area, the Health Service can help to give an insight into the complex mechanisms underlying accident involvement to enable an agenda for accident reduction to be agreed both by the community and by the professionals in the various agencies involved.

A common thread between these five groups is that, in general, they do not have more than a layman's knowledge of the accident problem, its underlying causes and what is currently being done in terms of engineering and education. Accident prevention does not feature as part of the training of these groups. Only by raising the awareness, competence and skills of these professionals will the full potential for accident prevention be realised. The task is too complex for any one agency to make a big improvement on its own and ways of working together should be sought as described in Chapter 4.

3. The NHS as an educator

The extent to which the NHS can and should fulfil these roles is determined in part by how much emphasis is put on road accidents being a public health issue in the same way as heart disease and smoking are seen to be.

(a) *Educating and training the professionals*

It has been suggested above that Health Service personnel in general have no more than a layman's knowledge of trends in accident occurrence or of progress in accident prevention work including education, training and publicity programmes. A priority must be to bring into the training of health professionals the basic skills to enable them to identify problems by analysing information from disparate sources, know who to go to for help to solve the problems, involve the community, help design and implement health promotion programmes and other countermeasures, and monitor and disseminate results to inform the community of progress in achieving objectives. This training will not only impart skills and knowledge but will also help to raise the status of safety both in the professions, then ultimately in the community. The HEA has a role to play in monitoring the content of, and updating where necessary, training packs for professionals such as the one developed for health visitors referred to in Chapter 4.

(b) *Education in schools*

Whilst consultation with the education service on all issues relating to education is important, the Health Education Authority has established a role within education through the health education input to personal and social education. Road safety is often already incorporated into materials the HEA produces. This is important as the health education component within the curriculum is highly regarded by educators. The TRRL study being carried out in Sheffield and Hertfordshire (Harland *et al.*, 1991) is demonstrating that health, education and highways departments can work together. At a local level there is great potential for these groups to devise interesting and relevant local examples for use in schools by teachers. At a national level the HEA has a role to play in devising educational materials for use in the school curriculum as well as in promoting safety as a public health issue to raise the profile both within the National Curriculum Council and with the public at large.

4. The role of the Director of Public Health

The Directors of Public Health (DPH) identify the health needs of the population; they are therefore centrally placed to highlight deficiencies and focus resources and programmes.

With the changes taking place within the Health Service, the DPH has the opportunity to influence the policies of the District Health Authority with respect to the prevention of children's road accidents. Many road accidents involving children are preventable and the WHO and Secretary of State for Transport's targets for casualty reduction are achievable. The Directors of Public Health have a central role to play by

- recognising in their annual reports that road accidents involving injury to children are a public health problem and that prevention is possible
- undertaking safety audits of contracts between the purchasing organisations and provider units to ensure that appropriate policies for accident prevention are included
- identifying research and training needs
- acting as a catalyst for local action both within the Health Service and between it and other agencies
- using influence to advocate a policy review within the District Health Authority with respect to standards of safety of carriage of children in cars by its own employees and encouraging high standards of driving through promotion of defensive driving schemes.

(a) Annual report of the Director of Public Health

Each year from 1990 each DPH has been required to publish a report which contains a health needs assessment. The DPH should be encouraged to provide accident data with an analysis that can inform the planning process for a child road accident prevention strategy for the District Health Authority. Progress towards achieving the objectives of this strategy can be monitored through the annual reports.

(b)   *Safety audit of contracts and service agreements*

One of the roles of the DPH is to review contracts and service agreements to ensure that the health of the population is being maintained and measures to improve it are being incorporated. If road accidents involving children are properly seen as a public health issue, the DPH could actively include the issue of safety by contracting with directly-managed units or Trusts for the provision of:

- computerised accident and emergency department records and a minimum set of data for accident prevention purposes, for routine surveillance and for informing decision making
- centres within the provider units that loan or sell safety aids such as baby car seats, child seats, cycle helmets, reflective items for bicycles and clothing, and books, games and videos with an accident prevention message,

and to ensure that

- maternity units and ante-natal clinics run, or have access to, baby seat loan schemes so that all babies have the opportunity to be carried safely from birth.

(c)   *Identifying research and training needs*

Resulting from the annual report and safety audit of contracts, the DPH is well placed to identify training needs for different groups within directly-managed units and Trusts and to advise FHSAs. If multi-agency working groups are to succeed, each group participating needs to be well informed about the accident prevention policies of the other groups and constraints on action. At the level of interface with the community, each group needs to be up to date about resources and initiatives.

At a broader level, the DPH should be in a position to identify research needs both within the Health Service and those more appropriately undertaken or funded by other agencies.

(d) Acting as a catalyst for local action

One of the main barriers to progress of local action is that there is no statutory requirement on health authorities for responsibility for co-ordination of co-operative working. Even when the DPH has identified areas for action, in the short term, it will still be down to the initiatives of local people. To this extent the DPH can act as a catalyst for action. The DPH can, in the annual report, identify other areas for action which are the responsibility of other agencies. For example, the DPH is being urged to include local policy and transport issues in the report whilst the local authorities are being asked to involve the health authority when drawing up their road safety plans. In the longer term it may even be possible for the DPH to consider the highway authority as a provider unit in terms of road safety provision for children.

(e) Developing health authority policy in respect of safety and driving standards of its own employees

The Local Authority Associations Road Safety Code of Good Practice urges local authorities to 'identify improvement targets for road accidents involving their own vehicles' and should encourage 'safe driving practices amongst all employees'. It further recommends that all vehicles owned or operated by the local authority should be 'maintained to the highest standards of safety and supplied with appropriate safety equipment' (paras 79–82).

Health authorities and NHS Trusts employ several thousand people across all grades from professional and managerial to ancillary staff. In any year, some will be involved in road traffic accidents during the course of their work, others will be involved in accidents outside of work. Some of these accidents will involve children. If health authorities across the country were to promote policies such as those recommended by the Local Authority Associations they would be setting an important example in accident prevention and making a contribution to a reduction in the numbers of road accidents involving children.

6 Pointers for Action

1. The Department of Health

Pressure for change has to come from the top down as well as from the bottom up. The Department of Health can take the lead by generally underlining that road accident prevention is part of health promotion, and specifically by:

- suggesting that action on road safety be included in the review process with Regional and District Health Authorities
- recognising road accidents as a public health issue and allocating resources for research and action, including commissioning the development of guidelines for good practice in multi-agency working to prevent road accidents
- considering, for the longer term, inter-departmental funding for road accident prevention work as it cuts across Health, Education and Science, and Transport. It should be recognised that the problem is too complex for single agency work at any level if a real impact is to be made towards achieving national and local targets
- considering applying pressure to clarify the lines of responsibility for child road accident prevention across government departments.

2. Regional Health Authorities

Action on Accidents (National Association of Health Authorities and RoSPA, 1990) lists ways in which Regional Heath Authorities can contribute towards accident prevention. In the context of road accidents involving children the RHA can collate and interpret accident statistics on a regional basis from information provided by the DHAs. The RHA can liaise with the Department of Transport at regional level and with groups of senior engineers from counties in the region to direct policy and set targets at this level. The RHA should encourage the DHA to set targets for accident reduction and support accident prevention work.

3. District Health Authorities, directly-managed units and NHS Trusts

There is a great deal of enthusiasm at the level of DHAs, directly-managed units and NHS Trusts and pressure for the following changes is coming from the various service units within the DHA:

- the Director of Public Health should have a central role in identifying needs and co-ordinating resources and programmes in accident prevention and health promotion activities related to accidents within the DHA
- the DHA's strategy should, where appropriate, include targets relating to accident prevention in its contracts with provider units. The DPH should monitor the contracts and undertake safety audits
- the DHA can, again through the contract procedure, require car seat loan schemes to be set up and administered by appropriate service units
- the DHA and provider units should formulate a policy for safe carriage of children by Health Service employees and encourage high standards of driving through the introduction of advanced and defensive driving courses
- the DHA, through the annual report of the DPH, should identify training needs for primary health care groups to enable them to gain an understanding of the child accident problem, how to respond to it and to develop skills needed for group working, especially at interagency level, as it is recognised that this will be difficult in the short term
- the DHA, through contracts and informed by the DPH, needs to define and put in place a strategy for action by the different groups, giving each one clear objectives and a remit for action. The DPH should collate information and monitor progress.

(a) Hospital units and Trusts

- the accident and emergency departments could provide health promotion literature and videos in waiting areas. This could be the same as, or similar to, material used by GPs. Suitable material needs to be developed
- in the hospitals, the accident and emergency departments

should be collecting information in a format that is useful to other service units and agencies

- hospitals, or other Health Service premises, could set up units for the sale or loan of safety equipment such as baby and child seats, cycle helmets, conspicuity aids, and literature, toys, games and videos, some of which need to be developed for this purpose.

(b) *Community health services, units and Trusts*

The groups considered here are health visitors, community nurses, midwives and the school health service. It is at this level that important work will be carried out and these groups need the commitment, guidance and support of the Department of Health through the Regional and District Health Authorities, and through the contracting process. These units can:

- monitor trends in accident occurrence to children whose health they are responsible for
- receive information from accident and emergency departments and GPs and pass information to the DPH and local highway authority
- encourage the use of cycle helmets and provide information on where to purchase them
- encourage the safe carriage of children in cars by setting up loan schemes or directing parents to existing schemes
- support initiatives sponsored by the local highway authority and act as a channel of communication
- help communities identify their road safety needs and help them communicate these to the local highway authority or other relevant agency
- support Traffic Clubs at all levels
- take opportunities as they arise for counselling parents and children.

4. Family Health Service Authorities and general practitioners

General practitioners hold an influential position and can continue to influence the community to help prevent road accidents to children. The GPs can support the DHA and can undertake all the action described above, with the addition of:

- taking opportunities to promote road safety for children through health promotion clinics
- providing interesting and relevant local material in waiting rooms. This material would be kept up to date by the health education units or the health promotion officer.

5. The Health Education Authority

Within its remit for education, the HEA should be considering:

- incorporating accident prevention programmes into its Strategic Plan
- working with other groups to initiate and support community projects which raise awareness and be exploring ways of getting the road safety message across to those most at risk
- using its contacts through the Health for All Network to disseminate information to other key agencies
- working with other groups to identify training and professional development requirements and jointly developing appropriate materials
- working to ensure that accident prevention features appropriately in relevant materials including those aimed at professionals who work with children with special educational needs
- where relevant consulting the Departments of Transport and Education and Science and national voluntary organisations, such as RoSPA, at the appropriate stages of curriculum development work
- liaising at a local level with health education units, highways departments and other groups so that material relevant to local problems can be produced for use by the community health services, FHSAs and hospital accident and emergency departments
- working with other agencies to develop innovative and effective materials such as toys, games and videos for use in waiting areas.

6. Conclusions

Initiatives aimed at reducing road accident involving children are many and varied, some are systematic and well researched, others are local projects with little institutional support. The cost of road accidents to the country and to individuals is high. There is no easy and inexpensive solution and many programmes under way at present will not yield quantifiable results for some time to come. The Health Service does have a role to play in reducing road accidents, some initiatives could be implemented now and others over the next few years. Although some of these initiatives may require new or redirected resources others can be incorporated into existing programmes.

Whilst it is recognised that there are many competing health demands at all levels, it is the Department of Health that sets priorities and has ultimate control over resources. *The Health of the Nation* has shown that the Department of Health (1991) *can* take the lead in recognising that road accidents *are* a health issue. What is needed now is the development of a policy framework for road accident prevention that will allow those in the health authorities to explore ways through their contract and service agreements to reduce injuries to the children for whose health they have responsibility. The Health Service has itself much to gain from fewer casualties resulting from road accidents.

References

Ampofo-Boateng, K. and Thomson, J. A. (1989) 'Child pedestrian accidents: a case for preventative medicine', *Health Education and Research*, 5(2), 265–74.

Ampofo-Boateng *et al.* 'A developmental and training study of children's ability to find safe routes to cross roads', to be published in *British Journal of Developmental Psychology*, **10**.

Antaki, C., Morris, P. E., and Flude, B. M. (1986) 'The effectiveness of the "Tufty Club" in road safety education', *British Journal of Educational Psychology*, **56**, 363–5.

Association of County Councils *et al.* (1989) *Local Authority Associations Road Safety Code of Good Practice*. Association of County Councils.

Benson, A. (1991) *Approaches to Local Child Accident Prevention Project*. Child Accident Prevention Trust.

Breeze, R. H. and Southall, D. (1990) *The Behaviour of Teenage Cyclists at T-junctions*. AA Foundation for Road Safety Research, Basingstoke.

British Institute for Traffic Education and Research (1990) *Secondary Steps*. BITER, Birmingham.

Carsten, O. M. J. *et al.* (1989) *Contributory Factors in Urban Traffic Accidents*. AA Foundation for Road Safety Research, Basingstoke.

Child Accident Prevention Trust (1989) *Basic Principles of Child Accident Prevention: a Guide to Action*. CAPT.

Child Accident Prevention Trust (1991) *Preventing Road Accidents to Children: a Training Resource for Health Visitors*. HEA.

Combes, G. (1991) *You Can't Watch Them Twenty-four Hours a Day: Parents' and Children's Perceptions, Understanding and Experience of Accidents and Accident Prevention*. CAPT, London.

Department of Health (1991) *The Health of the Nation: a Consultative Document for Health in England*. HMSO.

Department of Trade and Industry (1989) *Home and Leisure Accident Research, Eleventh Annual Report: Home Accident Surveillance System*. DTI.

Department of Transport (1987) *Road Safety: the Next Steps*. Department of Transport, London.

Department of Transport (1989) *Pedestrian Safety: New Proposals for Making Walking Safer*. Department of Transport.

Department of Transport (1990*a*) *Children and Roads: a Safer Way*. Department of Transport.

Department of Transport (1990*b*) *Road Accidents Great Britain 1989*. HMSO.

Department of Transport (1991) *Road Accidents Great Britain 1990*. HMSO.

Firth, D. E. (1973) *The Road Safety Aspects of the Tufty Club*, Department of the Environment: TRRL Laboratory Report LR604. Transport and Road Research Laboratory, Crowthorne.

General Accident, Department of Transport and Eastern Region County Councils (1990) *The Children's Traffic Club*. General Accident, Scotland.

Harland, D. J., Murray, G. and Tucker, S (1991) 'Road Safety Education; Making Safe Connections', proceedings from *Safety 91* J1–J9, Transport and Road Research Laboratory, Crowthorne.

Health Education Authority (1988) *Pregnancy Book*. HEA, London.

Health Education Authority (1989) *Birth to Five*. HEA.

Heraty, M. J. (1986) *Review of Pedestrian Safety Research*, Department of Transport: TRRL Contractor Report CR20. Transport and Road Research Laboratory, Crowthorne.

Institution of Highways and Transportation (1990) *Guidelines for Urban Safety Management*. IHT.

Lawson, S. D. (1990) *Accidents to Young Pedestrians: Distributions, Circumstances, Consequences and Scope for Countermeasures*. AA Foundation for Road Safety Research and Birmingham City Council. AA Foundation for Road Safety Research, Basingstoke.

McGarvie, A., Davies, R. F. and Sheppard, E. J. (1980) *A Study of Road Safety Film for Children*, Department of the Environment, Department of Transport: TRRL Research Report SR578. Transport and Road Research Laboratory, Crowthorne.

Mackie, A. M., Ward, H. A. and Walker, R. T. (1990) *Urban Safety Project 3: Overall Evaluation of Area Wide Schemes*, Department of Transport: TRRL Research Report RR263. Transport and Road Research Laboratory, Crowthorne.

Mills, P. J. (1989) *Pedal Cycle Accidents – a Hospital-based Study*,

Department of Transport: TRRL Research Report RR220. Transport and Road Research Laboratory, Crowthorne.

National Association of Health Authorities and Royal Society for the Prevention of Accidents (1990) *Action on Accidents: the Unique Role of the Health Service*. NAHA, Birmingham.

National Curriculum Council (1990) *Health Education* (Curriculum Guidance 5). NCC, York.

Road Safety and Design Partnership (1988) *The Nature of Children's Travel*. RSAD, Bristol.

Roberts, H. (1991) 'Accident prevention, a community approach', *Health Visitors* **64**(7), 219–20.

Rothengatter, T. and De Bruin, R. (eds.) (1988) *Road User Behaviour: Theory and Research*. Van Gorcum, Assen/ Maastricht, The Netherlands.

Royal Society for the Prevention of Accidents (1989) *Streets Ahead*. RoSPA, Birmingham.

Scottish Development Department (1989) *'Must do better': a Study of Child Pedestrian Accidents and Road Crossing Behaviour in Scotland*. Consultants' Report to Scottish Development Department by the MVA Consultancy. Scottish Office, Edinburgh.

Singh, A. (1982) 'Pedestrian Education', in Chapman, A. J., Wade, F. M. and Foot, H. C. (eds.) *Pedestrian Accidents*. Wiley, Chichester, pp. 71–108.

Singh, A. and Spear, M. (1989) *Traffic Education – a Survey of Current Provision and Practice in Secondary Schools*, Department of Transport: TRRL Contractor Report CR115. Transport and Road Research Laboratory, Crowthorne.

Singleton, W. and Woodcock, N. (1990) 'At terms with road safety in schools', *J. Traffic Med.*, **18**(2), 45–50.

Spear, M. and Singh, A. (1989) *Road Safety Education in Initial Teacher Training Programmes*, Department of Transport: TRRL Contractor Report CR117. Transport and Road Research Laboratory, Crowthorne.

Tight, M. R. (1987) 'Accident involvement and exposure to risk for children as pedestrians on urban roads.' PhD Thesis, University of London.

Towner, E. M. L. *et al.* (1990) 'Children and accidents: a survey of exposure to accident risk amongst schoolchildren', *Proceedings of Meeting of Society for Social Medicine*, Glasgow, September 1990 (unpublished).

Tunbridge, R. J. (1987) *The Use of Linked Transport – Health Road*

Casualty Data, Department of Transport: TRRL Research Report RR96. Transport and Road Research Laboratory, Crowthorne.

Tunbridge, R. J. *et al.* (1988) *An In-depth Study of Road Accident Casualties and their Injury Patterns*, Department of Transport: TRRL Research Report RR136. Transport and Road Research Laboratory, Crowthorne.

Tunbridge, R. J. *et al.* (1990) *Cost of Long-term Disability resulting from Road Traffic Accidents*, Department of Transport: TRRL Contractor Report CR212. Transport and Road Research Laboratory, Crowthorne.

Williams, T., Wetton, N. and Moon, A. (1990) *Health for Life: Health Education in the Primary School. A Teacher's Guide to Three Key Topics*, 2 volumes. Thomas Nelson, Walton on Thames.

APPENDIX 1

People consulted by the project

Gordon Avery — *Formerly Director of Public Health, South Warwickshire Health Authority*

Howard Baderman — *University College Hospital*

Malcolm Barrow — *Department of Trade and Industry*

Keith Belcher — *Department of Health*

Andy Benson — *Child Accident Prevention Trust*

Gill Combes — *Community Education Development Centre*

Margaret Connelly — *Nottingham County Council*

Andrew Clayton — *British Institute for Traffic Education and Research*

Jane Crofts — *County Road Safety Officer, Suffolk*

Andrew Crutchley — *Road Safety Officer, Birmingham City Council*

Charles Downing — *Transport and Road Research Laboratory*

John Drinkwater — *Department of Health*

Richard Evans — *Scottish Office*

Tony Greig — *Ludgershall Health Centre*

Phil Hanlon — *Greater Glasgow Health Board*

Gordon Harland — *Transport and Road Research Laboratory*

Jean Hopkin — *Transport and Road Research Laboratory*

John Howard — *Royal Society for the Prevention of Accidents*

Stephen Lawson	*City of Birmingham Engineers Department*
Sonya Leff	*Brighton Health Authority*
Mark McCarthy	*University College London, Community Medicine*
Colin McLennan	*Department of Transport*
Ros Meek	*Health Visitors' Association*
Paula Mills	*Transport and Road Transport Research Laboratory*
Brian Morrison	*Royal Society for the Prevention of Accidents*
Ann Mortlock	*County Road Safety Officer, Oxfordshire*
Margaret Noble	*Sheffield City Council/TRRL*
Charles Perryman	*Sheffield City Council*
Tom Pitcairn	*University of Edinburgh, Department of Psychology*
Lynn Richardson	*Nottinghamshire Family Health Service Authority*
Helen Roberts	*University of Glasgow, Department of Child Health and Obstetrics*
Amarjit Singh	*University of Reading, School of Education*
Terry Smith	*Road Safety Officer, Sheffield*
Bob Stone	*Transport and Road Research Laboratory*
David Stone	*University of Glasgow, Department of Child Health and Obstetrics*
Jimmy Thompson	*University of Strathclyde, Department of Psychology*
Gavin Thoms	*Sheffield Health Authority*

Liz Towner	*University of Newcastle upon Tyne, Department of Child Health*
Colin Tracey	*Former County Road Safety Officer, Essex*
Sean Walsh	*University of Newcastle upon Tyne, Department of Child Health*
Rosemary Welch	*County Road Safety Officer, Essex*
Diana Wilkinson	*Scottish Office*

Members of the Health Education Authority – Loraine Ashton, Lynda Finn

Members of the Prevention of Childhood Accidents Working Party, based at East Birmingham Health Authority

Members of Oxfordshire Health Authority joint working group

Group who attended one-day seminar at CAPT

Barbara Sabey	*Seminar chairman*
Gordon Avery	*South Warwickshire Health Authority*
Andy Benson	*Child Accident Prevention Trust*
Charles Downing	*Transport and Road Research Laboratory*
John Drinkwater	*Department of Health*
Karen Ford	*Health Education Authority*
Mike Hayes	*Child Accident Prevention Trust*
Hugh Jackson	*Child Accident Prevention Trust*
Christine McGuire	*Health Education Authority*
Philip Martin	*Department of Transport*
Brian Morrison	*Royal Society for the Prevention of Accidents*
Ann Mortlock	*Oxfordshire County Council Road Safety Officer*
Barry Pless	*Child Accident Prevention Trust*
Lynn Richardson	*Society of Health Education Officers*
Kevin Scott	*Department of Health*
Amarjit Singh	*University of Reading*
David Stone	*University of Glasgow*
Gavin Thoms	*Sheffield Health Authority*
Liz Towner	*University of Newcastle upon Tyne*
Sean Walsh	*University of Newcastle upon Tyne*
Heather Ward	*University College London*

Useful addresses and resources

The Health Education Authority
Hamilton House
Mabledon Place
London WC1H 9TX
(071-383 3833)

The Health Education Authority's Health Promotion
Information Centre has numerous resources lists, leaflets and
other material on many different health education topics,
including material for slow learners. It also has a
comprehensive selection of audio-visual material (for reference
only, which can be viewed at the centre between 9.00 am and
5.00 pm Monday to Friday).

Local contacts

Local health education/health promotion units

Each District Health Authority has its own health education/
health promotion unit, which carries stocks of all HEA leaflets/
posters and other information and resources. (Units should be
listed under the District Health Authority in the telephone
book: in case of difficulty, contact the HEA Liaison Section, or
the HEA Information Centre, at the address above.)

Local road safety officers

Each County Council, Metropolitan Borough Council and
London Borough Council employs road safety officers who are
responsible for education, training and publicity in relation to
road use and safety. Road safety officers work with schools and
help and support other professionals to incorporate road safety
in their work.

Road safety officers can usually be contacted through the
department responsible for highways.

National contacts

UK Health for All Network
PO Box 101
Liverpool L69 5BE
(051-231 1009)

The National Association of Health Authorities and Trusts
Chapter House
Chapter Street
London SW1
(071-233 7388)

The Health Visitors' Association and School Nurses Group
50 Southwark Street
London SE1
(071-387 7255)

The Department of Health
Wellington House
133–5 Waterloo Rd
London SE1 8UG
(071-972 2000)

The Health of the Nation, price £11.80, including postage and packing, is available from HMSO, PO Box 276, London SW8 5DT. (ISBN 0 10 1152329)

The Department of Transport
Room C17/08
2 Marsham Street
London SW1P 3EB
(071-276 6355)

Children and Roads: a Safer Way is available free of charge from the Department of Transport at the address above.

The Department of Education and Science
Elizabeth House
39 York Road
London SE1 7PH
(071-934 9000)

The Department of Trade and Industry
1–19 Victoria Street
London SW1
(071-215 5000)

British Institute of Traffic Education Research (BITER)
Kent House
Kent Street
Birmingham B5 6QF
(021-622 2402)

Association of County Councils
Eaton House
66a Eaton Square
London SW1W 9BH
(071-235 1200)

The Institution of Highways and Transportation
3 Lygon Place
Ebury Street
London SW1W 0JS
(071-730 5245)

Transport and Road Research Laboratory
Old Wokingham Road
Crowthorne
Berks RG11 6AU
(0344 773131)

AA Foundation for Road Safety Research
Fanum House
Basingstoke
Hants RG21 2EA
(0256 494604)

Children's Traffic Club
Suffolk County Council
Highways Dept
County Hall
Ipswich IP4 1LZ
(0473 230000)

Street-wise Kids
Parliament House
81 Black Prince Road
London SE1 1BP
(071-627 9618)

The Child Accident Prevention Trust (CAPT)
28 Portland Place
London W1N 4DE
(071-636 2545)

CAPT publishes an extensive list of materials and other information on child accident prevention. The CAPT library is open by appointment.

The Royal Society for the Prevention of Accidents (RoSPA)
Cannon House
The Priory Queensway
Birmingham B4 6BS
(021-200 2461)

RoSPA publishes a free catalogue of road safety resources and a bi-monthly paper *Care on the Road*.

'Play it Safe!' Campaign
Child Safety Campaign Headquarters
Room 606 Charitybase
The Chandlery
50 Westminster Bridge Road
London SE1 7QY
(071-721 7670)

The ALCAPP database is now based at the 'Play it Safe!' Campaign headquarters – the database also includes details of existing local child safety equipment loan schemes.

National Centre for Road Safety Education
Faculty of Education and Community Studies
University of Reading
Bulmershe Court
Reading RG6 1HY
(0734 318834/5)

The National Centre for Road Safety Education publishes three comprehensive lists of safety education resources, for ages 3–7, 7–11, and one for use in Secondary Schools which combines alcohol and safety education resources. All are available free by post. The centre welcomes visitors from 9.30 am to 3.30 pm Monday to Friday, and at other times by appointment.

Educational resources

The National Curriculum Council
Albion Wharf
25 Skeldergate
York YO1 2XL
(0904 622533)

TACADE (Teachers' Advisory Council on Alcohol and Drug Abuse)
3rd Floor
Furness House
Trafford Road
Salford
(061-848 0351)

TACADE publishes resource materials for schools on alcohol abuse.

Relevant Health Education Authority publications for schools

As well as resource lists on different topics, the Health Education Authority publishes books, research, teaching and training material on health education for use in schools and colleges. The following items contain sections on road safety and road accident prevention and may be of particular interest:

For primary schools

Health for Life by Trefor Williams, Noreen Wetton and Alysoun Moon.

Health for Life is a set of two teacher's guides on how to plan an overall health education strategy for primary schools:

Health for Life 1
Tackles a wide variety of themes that children need to understand in order to lead a healthy lifestyle. It includes photocopiable worksheets and action planners.

ISBN 0 17 423111 3
Price: £19.95

Health for Life 2
Provides an in-depth look at the key topics: 'The World of Drugs', 'Keeping Myself Safe' (which includes a section on road safety), 'Me and My Relationships'. It includes photocopiable worksheets and action planners.

ISBN 0 17 423113 X
Price: £29.95

Health for Life is available from:
Thomas Nelson & Sons Ltd
Nelson House
Mayfield Road
Walton on Thames
Surrey KT12 5PL

For secondary schools

Health and Self: Health Education in the Secondary School (1991)

Health and Self is a pack for teachers, based on Health Education 13–18, aimed at key stages 3 and 4. It includes three books for pupils and an introductory guide for teachers. One unit, 'Keeping Safe', looks at getting about, risks in general, and the subject of road safety. The first section of 'Keeping Safe' provides students with the opportunity to identify road traffic hazards that may occur on their way to school and discusses how they might cope with them.
Section Two encourages students to think about their own behaviour as pedestrians, identify the factors which affect the

way they cross roads and decide how they might reduce the risk to themselves.

The unit 'Coping with Accidents' allows students to explore what they understand by the term 'accident', and to identify the many factors involved. Other sections include activities to help students to identify ways of preventing accidents in the school environment, and to establish priorities for what to do at the scene of an accident.

Health and Self includes classroom activities and worksheets.

ISBN 0 901762 85 7
Price: £49.95
Available from:
Forbes Publications
2 Drayson Mews
London W8 4LY
(071-938 1035)

For 16- to 19-year-olds

Health Action Pack
A pack of health education material for use with 16- to 19-year-olds. Since young people in this age group have different health education needs the pack is designed to be highly flexible and can be adapted for different groups.

The pack contains a book – *Health Activities* – a photo pack, a games pack and background papers, including one on road safety, which looks at why 16- to 19-year-olds are particularly vulnerable road users.

A new edition is in preparation.

ISBN 0 86082 982 0
Price £39.95

Available from:
The Health Education Authority
Hamilton House
Mabledon Place
London WC1H 9TX
(071-383 3833)